CHRONIC LYMPHOCYTIC DIET COOKBOOK

Easy, Immune-Boosting Recipes, Foods, Nutritional Tips, Delicious Meals, And Guidelines For Optimal Health And Wellness – All You Need To Know

DR. AMARI VALERIE

TABLE OF CONTENTS

BONUS:

7 days meal plan recipes, ingredients, and detailed preparatory guidelines for Chronic Lymphocytic Leukemia

7 Desserts procedural recipes for Chronic Lymphocytic Leukemia and guidelines

7 Smoothies procedural recipes for Chronic Lymphocytic Leukemia and guidelines

DISCLAIMER

The information provided in this book, is for educational and informational purposes only and is not intended as medical advice. The content is not a substitute for professional medical advice, diagnosis, or treatment. Always seek the advice of your physician or other qualified health provider with any questions you may have regarding a medical condition. Never disregard professional medical advice or delay in seeking it because of something you have read in this book.

The dietary suggestions and recipes in this book are based on general guidelines and may not be suitable for everyone. Individual responses to foods can vary, and it is important to consult with a healthcare professional before making any significant changes to your diet.

The author and publisher of this book do not claim to cure or treat any medical condition. The information provided is based on research and personal experience and is intended to help readers make informed decisions about their diet and health.

Furthermore, I the author do not endorse any specific products, brands, treatments, or services that may be mentioned in this book. Any references to products, services, websites, or organizations are provided for informational purposes only and do not constitute an endorsement or recommendation by the author. The inclusion of such references does not imply any association, sponsorship, or affiliation between the author and the referenced entities.

The recipes and dietary suggestions in this book are designed to be safe and healthful. However, readers should use their own discretion and consult with a healthcare professional when necessary, especially if they have allergies, sensitivities, or other dietary restrictions.

ABOUT THIS BOOK

This "CHRONIC LYMPHOCYTIC DIET COOKBOOK" is an indispensable resource for those who are attempting to navigate the intricacies of Chronic Lymphocytic Leukemia (CLL). This comprehensive guide commences with a thorough examination of CLL, including its symptoms, diagnosis, and the critical role that diet plays in its management. It establishes a foundation for the necessity of a customized dietary approach by emphasizing the significance of nutrition for the immune system.

This book explores the necessity of key nutrients for immune health, the advantages of whole foods, and the importance of hydration, with an emphasis on immune-boosting principles. It promotes a comprehensive approach to the management of CLL through diet by instructing readers on the reduction of inflammatory foods and the creation of balanced meals.

This cookbook offers readership practical guidance on the establishment of realistic dietary objectives, the provisioning of a CLL-friendly larder, and the comprehension of portion sizes to facilitate the adoption of these dietary changes. It underscores the significance of interpreting and reading food labels, thereby empowering readers to make well-informed dietary decisions.

The culinary experience is further enhanced by this book's introduction of indispensable kitchen equipment and techniques. It encompasses essential kitchen equipment, fundamental culinary techniques for novices, and advice for the safe management of food. Furthermore, it provides readers with time-saving household techniques and advice on budget-friendly cooking, thereby ensuring that it is accessible to all.

This cookbook addresses common concerns and frequently asked questions, including whether diet can eradicate CLL and how to manage adverse effects through diet. It offers a comprehensive support system for individuals affected by CLL, including strategies for overcoming dietary restrictions, maintaining motivation on the diet plan, and locating support and resources.

This cookbook's chapters are meticulously crafted to accommodate a variety of dietary requirements and meal times. Breakfast recipes emphasize the significance of a nutritious start to the day, featuring protein-packed options, whole grain, fiber-rich, and anti-inflammatory ideas, as well as quick and simple smoothies.

Lunch recipes consist of lean protein options, healthy lipids, uncomplicated soups, immune-boosting salads and dressings, and balanced and portable options. Meal recipes for dinner prioritize the preparation of nutritious meals that include immune-boosting main dishes, vegetable-rich garnishes, one-pan meals that are effortless to prepare, and recipes for special occasions.

Healthy snacking suggestions, nutrient-dense ideas, rapid appetizers, homemade dips and spreads, and energy-boosting nibbles are all included in snack and appetizer recipes. Healthy sweet delights, low-sugar alternatives, fruit-based desserts, dairy-free alternatives, and straightforward pastry recipes comprise dessert recipes. Hydration, nutritious smoothies, herbal infusions, immune-boosting beverages, and the reduction of sugary beverages are all emphasized in beverage recipes.

With recipes that accommodate dietary allergies and intolerances, gluten-free and dairy-free alternatives, and vegan and vegetarian alternatives, special diet considerations are addressed. This book also provides readers with instructions on how to modify recipes to suit their specific requirements.

This cookbook contains a 7-day meal plan that is specifically designed for a chronic lymphocytic diet, and it includes detailed recipes, ingredients, and preparatory guidelines in addition to individual recipes. It also includes seven smoothie and dessert recipes, each with detailed procedural instructions.

Lastly, this book offers guidance on grocery shopping and meal planning, including strategies for reducing food waste, making a grocery list, wise shopping, bulk cooking, freezing meals, and creating a weekly meal plan. This comprehensive guide guarantees that readers receive complete assistance in their efforts to manage CLL by adhering to a nutritious and balanced diet.

CHAPTER ONE

Comprehending Chronic Lymphocytic Leukemia (CLL)

What is CLL? Chronic lymphocytic leukemia (CLL) is a form of malignancy that develops in the bone marrow and is characterized by excessive production of aberrant lymphocytes, a type of white blood cell. The normal cell function and immune response are disrupted by the accumulation of these malignant lymphocytes in the blood and bone marrow.

CLL is a disease that progresses slowly and is frequently identified in elderly individuals during routine blood tests before the onset of symptoms. Lifestyle modifications, targeted therapies, and regular monitoring are all essential components of effective CLL management.

Symptoms and Diagnosis Symptoms of CLL may be subtle and may include fatigue, enlarged lymph nodes, frequent infections, and unexplained weight loss. Blood tests that detect elevated lymphocyte levels, bone marrow biopsies, and imaging tests to assess lymph node enlargement are the standard diagnostic procedures. The management and treatment outcomes of CLL can be substantially influenced by early detection through routine medical check-ups. Consistent monitoring facilitates the tracking of disease progression and informs treatment decisions.

Diet is essential for the management of CLL, as it promotes overall health and improves the body's capacity to contend with treatment. A diet that is well-balanced and comprised of fruits, vegetables, lean proteins, and whole grains can assist in the maintenance of energy levels, the enhancement of immune function, and the mitigation of treatment-related adverse effects. Patients are frequently advised to restrict their intake of processed foods, fructose, and saturated fats, while simultaneously maintaining a healthy weight and remaining hydrated. Dietary plans can be customized to meet the unique requirements and preferences of each individual by consulting with a dietitian.

The immune system is significantly bolstered by proper nutrition, which is especially crucial for those with CLL. Leafy greens, berries, nuts, seeds, and oily fish are examples of nutrient-rich foods that are essential for the maintenance of immune defenses. These foods are rich in vitamins, minerals, and antioxidants. Zinc, vitamin D, vitamin C, and probiotics are particularly advantageous for immune function. The body's resistance to infections and overall health can be improved by incorporating a diverse array of these nutrients into daily meals.

Practical Illustrations:

• Balanced Diet: Incorporate a diverse array of fruits and vegetables (such as citrus, berries, and carrots) into each meal.

• Hydration: Aim to consume a minimum of eight containers of water each day to facilitate bodily functions and mitigate treatment-related adverse effects.

• Lean Proteins: Incorporate sources such as chicken, fish, lentils, and legumes to ensure that the body receives the necessary proteins without accumulating excess fat.

• Whole Grains: To ensure consistent energy levels, choose whole wheat bread, quinoa, and brown rice.

• Reducing the Consumption of Processed Foods: Opt for healthier alternatives, such as nuts and fresh fruit, rather than munchies that are high in sugar and sodium.

Individuals with CLL can enhance their quality of life and more effectively manage their condition by incorporating these dietary habits.

The Fundamentals Of An Immune-Boosting Diet

An immune-boosting diet emphasizes the integration of a diverse array of nutrients that bolster the immune system. This encompasses a well-rounded diet that includes fruits, vegetables, whole cereals, lean proteins, and healthy lipids. For example, a typical meal might consist of grilled salmon with sautéed broccoli for dinner, a quinoa and vegetable salad for lunch, and a spinach and berry smoothie for breakfast. The objective is to ingest foods that are abundant in minerals such as selenium and zinc, as well as vitamins A, C, D, and E, which are essential for immune function.

Key Nutrients For Immune Health

Certain nutrients are essential for the preservation of a robust immune system. The production of white blood cells is facilitated by vitamin C, which is present in citrus fruits, strawberries, and bell peppers.

The immune response is influenced by vitamin D, which is obtainable through fortified dairy products and sunlight exposure. Zinc, which is found in almonds, seeds, and legumes, is essential for the proper functioning of immune cells.

Selenium, which is present in Brazil nuts and seafood, is beneficial in the prevention of cellular injury. By incorporating these nutrients into a varied diet, your body is better prepared to combat maladies.

Advantages Of Whole Foods

Minimally processed whole foods, including fruits, vegetables, whole cereals, and lean proteins, are abundant in essential nutrients and fiber. For instance, selecting an apple over apple juice preserves fiber and minimizes added carbohydrates, which aids in the regulation of blood sugar levels and the preservation of a healthy digestive system. Antioxidants and phytochemicals are also present in whole foods, which are beneficial to the immune system. By substituting processed treats with nuts, seeds, or fresh produce, one can substantially improve their overall health.

The Significance Of Hydration

It is essential to maintain proper hydration to maintain immune health, as water is essential for all physiological functions, including the production of lymph, which transports white blood cells and other immune system cells. Aim to consume a minimum of eight 8-ounce glasses of water each day. Green tea, which is rich in antioxidants, is an example of a herbal beverage that can also contribute to your fluid intake. Maintaining optimal hydration levels can be achieved by setting reminders to consume throughout the day and keeping a reusable water container readily available.

Reducing The Consumption Of Inflammatory Foods

To bolster your immune system, it is crucial to limit your consumption of inflammatory foods, including refined carbohydrates, processed foods, and trans fats. For instance, choosing whole-grain bread over white bread and substituting sugary beverages with water or green tea can decrease inflammation in the body. These dietary modifications alleviate the stress on your immune system and aid in the prevention of chronic inflammation, which is associated with a variety of diseases.

Formulating Well-Balanced Meals

To guarantee sustained energy and nutrient intake, it is necessary to combine proteins, healthful lipids, and carbohydrates in appropriate proportions. This is the process of preparing balanced meals.

For example, a nutritious plate could consist of a mixed green salad with an olive oil vinaigrette, seared chicken (protein), and roasted sweet potatoes (carbohydrates). The plate method, which involves filling half of your plate with vegetables, a quarter with protein, and a quarter with whole carbohydrates, can facilitate meal planning and guarantee that you are consuming a diverse array of nutrients at each meal.

CHAPTER TWO

Commencing Your Dietary Plan

Consult with a healthcare provider or dietitian who is knowledgeable about Chronic Lymphocytic Leukemia (CLL) to begin. They can customize a diet plan to meet the specific health requirements of each individual.

Concentrate on a diet that is well-balanced and contains a variety of fruits, vegetables, lean proteins, and whole cereals. For instance, breakfast could consist of oatmeal with berries and a sprinkling of almonds, lunch could be a quinoa salad with grilled chicken and mixed greens, and supper could be steamed salmon with a side of roasted vegetables. Aim for a diet that is high in nutrients and limited in processed foods to promote overall health and well-being.

Establishing Practical Dietary Objectives

Begin by setting modest, feasible objectives, such as substituting sweetened beverages with water or including an additional serving of vegetables in each meal. For example, if you consume vegetables only once per day, strive to incorporate them into two meals per day. Maintaining motivation can be facilitated by celebrating minor victories and monitoring your progress. It is simpler to maintain your new dietary habits in the long term when you implement gradual changes, as they are more sustainable.

Creating A Pantry That Is CLL-Friendly

Maintaining a nutritious diet necessitates a well-stocked larder. Incorporate a diverse array of seasonings, canned legumes, low-sodium broths, and whole grains (e.g., quinoa and brown rice).

Healthy lipids, such as olive oil and nuts, lean proteins like chicken breast and tofu, and fresh and frozen fruits and vegetables should also be included as essentials. Preparing nutritious dishes without the use of commercial foods is facilitated by the availability of these ingredients.

Tips For Meal Planning And Preparation

Preparing dishes for the upcoming week is crucial for maintaining a nutritious diet. Begin by formulating a menu that encompasses a diverse selection of foods from all food categories. Prepare dishes in advance to save time during the week, such as baking a quantity of chicken breasts or preparing a large pot of vegetable soup.

Store pre-prepared meals and ingredients in hermetic containers to facilitate the rapid assembly of nutritious dishes.

This method mitigates the incentive to select less nutritious convenience foods.

Comprehension Of Portion Sizes

It is essential to employ portion control to sustain a nutritious diet. Visual aids can be employed to assist in the determination of appropriate portion proportions.

A protein serving should be approximately the size of your palm, a cereal serving should fit into your cupped hand, and vegetables should occupy at least half of your plate.

Accurate portion measurements can also be achieved through the use of measuring instruments, such as a kitchen scale and cups. Preventing excess and enhancing the management of one's nutritional consumption are facilitated by being mindful of portions.

Acquiring the ability to comprehend food labels can assist you in making more nutritious decisions. Begin by verifying the quantity of servings per container and the dimensions of each serving.

Examine the calories and be mindful of the quantities of added sugars, sodium, and saturated fat. The fewer ingredients and the more recognizable they are, the better. Ingredients are enumerated in descending order by weight.

For instance, opt for whole grain bread that is labeled with the term "whole grain" as its initial ingredient, as opposed to a product that contains an extensive list of unfamiliar additives.

CHAPTER THREE

Kitchen Tools And Techniques That Are Essential

Essential Household Appliances

Beginners should concentrate on the most fundamental kitchen equipment, including a chef's knife, cutting board, measuring cups and utensils, a skillet, and a saucepan, to efficiently set up a kitchen.

Additionally, it is essential to have a dependable blender or food processor, a robust mixing basin, and a spatula. These tools allow you to effortlessly prepare a diverse array of recipes, including the precise measurement of ingredients and the slicing of vegetables, as well as the blending of soups and beverages.

Fundamental Culinary Methods For Novices

Begin with the most basic culinary skills, including slicing, sautéing, simmering, and baking. For instance, practice the following: finely chopping scallions for a variety of dishes, sautéing vegetables in olive oil until they are tender, boiling pasta to the ideal al dente, and baking poultry until it is juicy and golden. A solid foundation for more complex formulas is established by mastering these techniques.

Tips For The Secure Handling Of Food

To prevent cross-contamination, it is imperative to cleanse your hands before cooking and after handling raw flesh. Utilize distinct cutting boards for vegetables and uncooked meat. Ensure that your kitchen surfaces are clean, perishable items are promptly refrigerated, and meat is cooked to the recommended internal temperature using a food thermometer. These procedures guarantee food safety and mitigate the likelihood of contaminated ailments.

Kitchen Shortcuts That Save Time

By preparing ingredients in abundance, such as chopping a week's worth of vegetables in one session and preserving them in airtight containers, you can save time. Cook dishes with minimal effort by employing kitchen appliances such as an Instant Pot or slow cooker. Freeze portions of prepared dishes for convenient reheating on days when one is in a hurry. These techniques simplify the culinary process and enhance the efficiency of meal preparation.

Budget-Friendly Cooking

Arrange your meals with the seasonal produce and promotions at your neighborhood grocery store. When feasible, purchase in volume and select store brands to reduce expenses. Extend your budget by integrating affordable staples such as rice, pasta, and legumes into your meals. Creatively repurpose leftovers by transforming them into new dishes to reduce waste and optimize value.

Common Questions And Concerns

However, diet is essential for the management of symptoms and the improvement of quality of life, even though Chronic Lymphocytic Leukemia (CLL) cannot be cured. There is a common misconception among patients that certain foods can cure the disease.

However, the emphasis should be on a well-balanced diet that is abundant in fruits, vegetables, lean proteins, and whole cereals to support overall health and immunity. For example, the inclusion of foods that are rich in antioxidants, such as verdant greens and berries, can effectively mitigate oxidative stress, which is advantageous for patients with chronic lymphocytic leukemia.

Is It Possible To Cure CLL Through Diet?

No, diet alone is not capable of curing CLL; however, it can provide substantial assistance in its management. Proper nutrition is beneficial for the immune system, helps maintain stamina, and can alleviate some of the adverse effects of treatment. For instance, consuming a diet that is abundant in vitamins and minerals can enhance your body's resilience and its ability to respond to both the disease and its treatments.

Dietary Modifications For The Management Of Side Effects

Common adverse effects of CLL treatment, including fatigue, vertigo, and appetite loss, can be mitigated through diet modification. Staying hydrated, consuming small, frequent meals, and incorporating ginger or peppermint can all assist in the reduction of nausea. Furthermore, foods that are rich in protein and healthy lipids, such as avocados and almonds, can offer long-term energy and alleviate fatigue. Smoothies and soups may be more convenient to ingest during periods of diminished appetite.

Dealing With Dietary Restrictions

Careful planning is necessary to navigate dietary restrictions, whether they are the result of pre-existing conditions or treatment. For instance, if certain foods, such as those that are high in fiber, cause gastrointestinal distress during chemotherapy, substitute them with softer, blander options, such as rice, bananas, and applesauce.

It is imperative to seek the advice of a dietitian to develop a customized plan that meets nutritional requirements while also accommodating these constraints.

Maintaining Your Motivation For Your Diet Plan

It can be difficult to maintain motivation while adhering to a diet plan; however, establishing modest, feasible objectives can be beneficial. Celebrate accomplishments, such as achieving a hydration goal or attempting a new, nutritious recipe.

Enrolling in a support group, whether it be in-person or online, can offer accountability and motivation. Additionally, maintaining a food diary can assist in monitoring progress and making necessary adjustments.

Locating Assistance And Resources

It is essential to locate support and resources to sustain a healthful diet while living with CLL. For moral support and guidance, consult healthcare providers, dietitians, and patient support groups. Recipes, meal plans, and forums are frequently accessible through online platforms and community resources, where patients can exchange insights and experiences. By utilizing these resources, you can receive both emotional support and practical advice during your dietary voyage.

CHAPTER FOUR

Breakfast Recipes

To provide your body and mind with the necessary energy, begin your day with a nutritious breakfast. Examples include a slice of whole-grain toast with avocado and a poached egg, or a serving of Greek yogurt garnished with fresh berries and a drizzle of honey. These alternatives offer a well-balanced combination of carbohydrates, protein, and healthful lipids.

The Significance Of A Nutritious Breakfast

It is imperative to consume a nutritious breakfast to sustain one's energy and concentration throughout the day. It is beneficial for the regulation of blood sugar levels and the stimulation of the metabolism. For example, a breakfast that includes oatmeal, almonds, and fruits can enhance cognitive function and provide sustained energy.

Smoothie Recipes That Are Quick And Simple

Smoothies are a convenient and efficient method of introducing nutrients into the body. For a nutritious and delectable green smoothie, combine a banana, a fistful of spinach, a scoop of protein powder, and almond milk. Alternatively, for a revitalizing start, combine frozen berries, Greek yogurt, and a small amount of citrus juice.

Breakfast Options That Are High In Protein

By incorporating protein into your breakfast, you can maintain muscle mass and remain satisfied for an extended period. Consider a quinoa dish with poached egg and avocado segments, or scrambled eggs with spinach and feta cheese. These dishes are effortless to prepare and offer a substantial quantity of protein to kickstart your day.

Breakfasts That Are High In Fiber And Whole Grains

Fiber and whole grains are essential for the regulation of blood sugar levels and the maintenance of digestive health. Choose a whole-grain muffin with flaxseeds or a bowl of steel-cut oats garnished with blueberries and chia seeds. These alternatives are not only satisfying, but they also contribute to the preservation of a healthy intestine.

Anti-Inflammatory Breakfast Ideas

Chronic inflammation can be mitigated and overall health can be enhanced by consuming an anti-inflammatory brunch. Consider a chia seed pudding made with almond milk, garnished with fresh berries and a sprinkle of cinnamon, or a smoothie that includes pineapple, ginger, and turmeric. These ingredients possess inherent anti-inflammatory properties that contribute to your overall health.

Lunch Recipes

These balanced and portable concepts can simplify the process of preparing meals. Choose a whole grain wrap that is stuffed with lean turkey or poultry, as well as a variety of vegetables such as cucumbers, tomatoes, and lettuce. For an extra burst of flavor and healthy lipids, add a spread of avocado or hummus.

An additional alternative is a quinoa salad that is brimming with vibrant vegetables, including broccoli, carrots, and bell peppers and is garnished with broiled salmon or tofu for protein. For a meal that is both fast and satisfying, prepare a quantity of vegetable soup with low-sodium broth. For an additional source of protein and fiber, incorporate beans or lentils.

Salads And Dressings That Enhance Immunity

Enhance your immune system by consuming salads that are rich in nutrients and homemade dressings. Begin by building a foundation of verdant greens, such as spinach or kale, and subsequently incorporate immune-boosting ingredients, including berries, bell peppers, and citrus fruits.

For a satisfying supper, add lean protein, such as grilled chicken or chickpeas. To create a homemade vinaigrette, combine olive oil, lemon juice, garlic, and herbs such as oregano or basil. This healthful and flavorful option will improve the taste of your salad while also replenishing essential nutrients.

Lunch Options With Lean Protein

It is imperative to include lean protein in your lunch to preserve muscle health and sustain energy levels. Choose either grilled chicken breast, turkey, or fish such as salmon or tuna as your primary protein source. For a well-rounded entrée, serve it with a side of steamed vegetables or a verdant green salad. Tofu, tempeh, lentils, and legumes are exceptional plant-based sources of protein that can be incorporated into salads, wraps, or stir-fries to provide a satisfying meal option for vegetarians or vegans.

Incorporating Nutritious Fats

Brain function, hormone production, and overall health are all dependent on the consumption of healthy lipids. Incorporate sources of healthy fats into your supper to promote optimal well-being and feel satiated. Sprinkle nuts and seeds on top of your broth or salad, drizzle olive oil over roasted vegetables, or add avocado segments to your sandwich or salad. Not only do these straightforward additives improve the flavor and texture of your meal, but they also supply essential nutrients such as vitamin E and omega-3 fatty acids.

Soups That Are Both Simple And Satisfying

Soups are a nourishing and comforting lunch option, particularly during the harsher months. For a nutritious and satisfying meal, prepare a quantity of homemade broth that includes a variety of vegetables, beans, and whole cereals. Select soups that are broth-based rather than creamy to regulate your calorie and fat intake. Try out various flavor combinations, such as vegetable curry broth with lentils and coconut milk or minestrone with whole-grain pasta and white beans. For a brunch that is both substantial and comprehensive, serve it with a side of whole-grain bread or crackers.

Dinner Recipes

Dinner can be an opportunity for individuals who adhere to a chronic lymphocytic diet to concentrate on nutrient-dense meals that promote overall health. Consider implementing lean proteins, such as grilled chicken or fish, in conjunction with whole cereals, such as brown rice or quinoa.

It is advisable to include a diverse array of vegetables on your plate to guarantee that you are consuming a diverse array of vitamins and minerals. To maintain interest, consider incorporating various cuisines, such as preparing a substantial lentil broth or a vegetable stir-fry with tofu. By prioritizing wholesome ingredients and a variety of flavors, it is possible to prepare meals that are both nourishing and immune-boosting.

Planned Dinners: It is beneficial to organize your meals in advance to guarantee that they are nutritious and well-balanced. Begin by compiling a list of protein sources, including tofu, poultry, or legumes, and incorporating them into your weekly menu. Aim to fill half of your plate with colorful produce by pairing these with a variety of vegetables. Be sure to include whole grains and nutritious lipids, such as avocado or olive oil, to complete your meal.

To maintain the level of excitement, experiment with various culinary methods and flavor combinations. With a little forethought, it is possible to prepare nutritious dinners that promote your overall well-being.

Main Dishes that Support Immunity: When emphasizing immune support, it may be advantageous to incorporate specific foods into your main dishes. Garlic, ginger, turmeric, and verdant greens like spinach or kale are all ingredients that are high in vitamins and antioxidants.

Consider preparing soups or stews that are rich in immune-boosting ingredients, such as chicken, legumes, and vegetables. Furthermore, incorporate lean protein sources, such as salmon or lean portions of meat, to ensure that the body receives the necessary nutrients for immune function.

By selecting primary dishes that emphasize immune support, you can contribute to the enhancement of your body's natural defenses and the promotion of overall health.

Vegetable-Rich Side Dishes: Side dishes are an exceptional opportunity to integrate a diverse array of vegetables into your meals. Opt for colorful options such as broccoli, carrots, and bell peppers, which are abundant in antioxidants, minerals, and vitamins. To preserve the nutrients and natural characteristics of vegetables, it is advisable to roast or sauté them. To improve the flavor of your side dishes without resorting to heavier condiments or dressings, experiment with various herbs and seasonings. Filling your plate with vegetable-rich sides can enhance your overall health, support digestion, and increase your fiber intake.

Simple One-Pan Meals: For individuals who are occupied and adhere to a chronic lymphocytic diet, one-pan meals can be a godsend. These straightforward dishes are ideal for busy weeknights, as they necessitate minimal preparation and cleaning. Begin by selecting a protein source, such as chicken, tofu, or seafood, and combining it with a variety of vegetables, including scallions, zucchini, and bell peppers. Combine all ingredients with your preferred herbs and seasonings, and then roast or stir-fry until fully cooked.

One-pan dishes are not only convenient, but they also enable the creation of an infinite number of flavor combinations and customizations. By mastering a few go-to recipes, you can simplify the meal prep process and enjoy delectable, nutritious meals with simplicity.

CHAPTER FIVE

Recipes For Snacks And Appetizers

Focus on nutrient-dense nibbles and canapés that are high in fiber and low in sugar when it comes to a chronic lymphocytic diet. Consider preparing vegetable sticks with hummus, homemade guacamole with whole grain crackers, or Greek yogurt with assorted fruit. These alternatives offer a harmonious combination of protein, healthy lipids, and carbohydrates to maintain your energy levels in between meals and promote your overall health.

Healthy Snacking Advice: Whenever feasible, choose whole foods, including fruits, vegetables, nuts, and seeds, over-processed munchies. To prevent overheating, it is crucial to pre-portion foods into tiny containers or packages. Portion control is essential.

Additionally, refrain from snacking unless you are genuinely ravenous, rather than out of habit or boredom, and pay attention to your body's hunger signals.

Nutrient-dense Snack Ideas: To guarantee that you are consuming a diverse array of vitamins and minerals, incorporate a variety of nutrient-dense foods into your snacking. Kale chips sprinkled with nutritional yeast for a cheesy flavor, apple slices with almond butter for a satisfying crunch and a dose of healthy fats, or a small sprinkling of mixed nuts and dried fruit for a fast energy boost are some ideas.

Quick and Easy canapés: Prepare straightforward canapés that are both nutritious and time-saving. Options such as cucumber slices garnished with tuna salad, whole grain pita chips with roasted red pepper hummus, or cherry tomatoes filled with herbed goat cheese should be taken into account. These appetizers are not only delectable, but they also offer a well-balanced combination of macronutrients that will leave you feeling full.

Homemade Dips and Spreads: By preparing your dips and spreads, you can maintain control over the ingredients and avoid the added carbohydrates and preservatives that are present in store-bought versions.

Attempt to create a velvety hummus by combining chickpeas, tahini, lemon juice, garlic, and olive oil. Alternatively, create a flavorful guacamole by combining avocado, lime juice, cilantro, and jalapeno.

For a nutritious and satisfying appetizer or refreshment, serve these dips with whole grain crackers or raw vegetable spears.

Recipes For Beverages

Using fresh, whole ingredients is essential for the production of beverages that promote health and wellness. For instance, a straightforward yet potent immune-boosting beverage can be prepared by combining one cup of freshly strained orange juice, half a teaspoon of grated ginger, and a tablespoon of honey. In addition to the antimicrobial benefits of honey and the anti-inflammatory properties of ginger, this combination is a rich source of vitamin C. Experiment with a variety of fruits, herbs, and seasonings to produce nutritious and delicious beverages that are tailored to your health requirements and flavor preferences.

Hydration And Immune System Function

It is essential to maintain a healthy immune system by staying hydrated, as water assists in the transportation of nutrients to cells and the elimination of contaminants from the body. Aim to consume a minimum of eight 8-ounce glasses of water per day, with an additional eight glasses if you are physically active or reside in a humid climate. Enhance the flavor and health benefits of your water by incorporating slices of cucumber, mint, or lemon. Coconut water and herbal infusions are also viable alternatives to ordinary water, as they provide both hydration and supplementary nutrients.

Recipes For Nutritious Smoothies

Nutritious smoothies are an excellent method for incorporating a significant amount of vitamins and minerals into a meal that is both convenient and simple to consume. Begin by incorporating a cup of frozen berries, half a banana, a teaspoon of protein powder, and a tablespoon of chia seeds into a base of verdant greens such as spinach or kale. Combine these ingredients with one cup of almond milk or any other plant-based milk to create a nutritious and delectable smoothie. This combination is crucial for the maintenance of overall health and vitality, as it contains antioxidants, fiber, protein, and healthy lipids.

Infusions And Teas Of Herbal Origin

In addition to providing a soothing effect, herbal beverages, and infusions can also provide a variety of health benefits. For example, ginger tea has the potential to alleviate inflammation and improve digestion, while chamomile tea is recognized for its soothing properties and can promote better sleep.

Steep a small quantity of fresh or dried herbs, such as rosemary, lavender, or mint, in boiling water for 5-10 minutes to create a straightforward herbal infusion. Consider incorporating a small amount of honey or citrus into these teas to enhance their flavor and health benefits. The teas can be enjoyed either warm or cooling.

Homemade Immune-Boosting Drinks

The preparation of homemade immune-boosting beverages can be both straightforward and delectable. A favored recipe involves the addition of a sprinkle of turmeric, a teaspoon of apple cider vinegar, half a cup of green tea, and half a cup of pomegranate juice. Antioxidants, vitamins, and anti-inflammatory compounds are abundant in this beverage, which promotes immune function. Drink this mixture daily, particularly during the cold and flu season, to fortify your body's inherent defenses.

Reducing Sugary Beverages

It is imperative to decrease the consumption of saccharine beverages to preserve one's health, as excessive sugar consumption can result in a variety of health complications, such as diabetes and obesity. Substitute sugary sodas and energy beverages with healthier alternatives, such as homemade fruit-infused water, herbal teas, or sparkling water with a dash of natural fruit juice. By reducing your consumption of sugary beverages, you can improve your overall health and reduce your calorie intake, resulting in improved weight management and a reduced risk of chronic diseases.

CHAPTER SIX

Special Dietary Requirements

It is imperative to maintain a balanced diet for individuals diagnosed with chronic lymphocytic leukemia (CLL). This encompasses the inclusion of nutrient-dense foods, such as fruits, vegetables, whole cereals, and lean proteins. It is imperative to refrain from consuming processed foods, excessive carbohydrates, and unhealthy lipids.

For instance, a meal could include grilled chicken breast, a quinoa salad with mixed greens, and a side of steamed broccoli.

Furthermore, it is essential to maintain hydration by consuming an adequate amount of water and to restrict alcohol consumption to promote overall health and alleviate symptoms.

Managing Food Allergies And Intolerances

Careful menu planning and label reading are essential for managing food allergies and intolerances to prevent the consumption of triggering ingredients. For example, individuals with gluten intolerance must refrain from consuming wheat-based products and instead choose gluten-free cereals such as rice, quinoa, or maize. It is essential to familiarize oneself with the most prevalent allergens in processed foods and read the ingredient lists. Frequently, the most secure method is to prepare meals at home, where you can regulate the ingredients.

Recipes That Are Free Of Gluten

The process of developing gluten-free recipes can be both straightforward and delectable when the appropriate substitutions are made. For breakfast, contemplate a smoothie bowl that is garnished with almonds and seeds and is composed of blended fruits and gluten-free cereals. Dinner may consist of a baked salmon filet served with roasted sweet potatoes and asparagus, while lunch may consist of a quinoa salad with assorted vegetables and a lemon-tahini vinaigrette. By employing inherently gluten-free ingredients, you can savor a diverse selection of nutritious and flavorful dishes.

Dairy-Free Substitutes

For individuals who refrain from consuming dairy, numerous alternatives can be seamlessly incorporated into their diet. Substitute almond, soy, or oat milk for cow's milk in your morning cereal or coffee. Incorporate coconut yogurt into your smoothies and salads, and experiment with dairy-free cheese prepared from cashews or soy for your sandwiches and pizzas. For example, a dairy-free lasagna could be prepared by layering gluten-free noodles with a flavorful tomato sauce made with vegetables and cashew cheese.

Vegetarian And Vegan Alternatives

A well-planned vegan or vegetarian diet can supply all of the essential nutrients. Incorporate a diverse array of plant-based proteins, such as chickpeas, lentils, tempeh, and tofu. For a nutritious meal, consider a lentil stew that is served over brown rice or quinoa and contains an abundance of vegetables. Hummus with carrot spears or a handful of assorted nuts are potential snacks. Your nutritional requirements will be met by consuming a variety of fruits, vegetables, cereals, and legumes.

Modifying Recipes To Meet Specific Requirements

Altering recipes to accommodate specific dietary requirements necessitates the substitution of ingredients without sacrificing flavor. Consider using a flaxseed meal mixed with water as a vegan substitute for eggs in a recipe. Garlic, rosemary, and lemon juice are effective herbs and seasonings for reducing sodium and enhancing flavor. For instance, a cauliflower crust could be utilized to create a gluten-free, low-sodium pizza that is garnished with a variety of vegetables, dairy-free cheese, and fresh tomato sauce.

CHAPTER SEVEN

Seven Days Meal Plan Recipes, Ingredients, And Detailed Preparatory Guidelines For The Chronic Lymphocytic Diet

DAY ONE:

Breakfast: Quinoa Breakfast Bowl

• **INGREDIENTS:**

o One cup of prepared quinoa

o 1/2 cup of almond milk

o 1/4 cup of assorted fruit

o One tablespoon of honey

o One tablespoon of minced nuts (such as almonds, walnuts, or pecans)

• *PREPARATION:*

1. Combine almond milk with prepared quinoa in a basin.

2. Sprinkle chopped almonds, honey, and a variety of fruit on top.

Mediterranean Chickpea Salad for Lunch

• **INGREDIENTS:**

o One can of legumes, drained and rinsed

o One cup of cherry tomatoes, halved

o Diced cucumber, 1/2

o One-quarter cup of finely sliced red onion

o Two tablespoons of olive oil

o One tablespoon of lemon juice

o 1/4 cup of shredded feta cheese (optional)

• PREPARATION:

1. Chickpeas, cucumber, cherry tomatoes, and red onion should be combined in a sizable basin.

2. Drizzle with lemon juice and olive oil, and then swirl to combine.

3. If desirable, garnish with feta cheese.

Dinner: Baked Salmon with Asparagus

• INGREDIENTS:

o Two salmon fillets

o One bundle of asparagus

o Two tablespoons of olive oil

o One lemon, cut

o Add salt and pepper to taste

• *PREPARATION:*

1. Preheat the oven to 400°F (200°C).

2. Arrange asparagus and salmon fillets on a baking tray.

3. Season with salt and pepper and drizzle with olive oil.

4. Arrange lemon segments on top of the salmon.

5. Bake for 12-15 minutes until the asparagus is tender and the salmon is fully cooked.

Snack:

• Hummus-topped carrot spears.

Juice:

• Kale and Green Apple Juice

DAY TWO:

Breakfast: Avocado Toast

• INGREDIENTS:

o Two slices of whole-grain bread

o One mature avocado

o Add salt and pepper to taste

o Red pepper granules (optional)

• *PREPARATION:*

1. Toast the bread segments until they are a golden brown color.

2. Spread the avocado evenly on the toast by mashing it.

3. If desired, add salt, pepper, and red pepper flakes.

• INGREDIENTS:

o One cup of prepared quinoa

o One roasted chicken breast, divided

o. Half a cup of cherry tomatoes

O 1/4 cup of finely sliced cucumber

o Two tablespoons of balsamic vinaigrette

o Garnish with fresh basil fronds

• *PREPARATION:*

1. Cooked quinoa, cherry tomatoes, cucumber, and seared chicken should be combined in a bowl.

2. Drizzle the balsamic vinaigrette over the salad and toss to incorporate.

3. Add fresh basil leaves as a garnish.

• INGREDIENTS:

o One cup of drained dried legumes

o One diced onion

o Two carrots, cut

o Two minced celery stalks

o Four pints of vegetable broth

o One teaspoon of dried thyme

o Add salt and pepper to taste

• *PREPARATION:*

1. Sauté celery, carrots, and onion in a substantial saucepan until they are tender.

2. Incorporate dried thyme, vegetable bouillon, and lentils.

3. Bring the mixture to a boil, then reduce the heat and allow it to simmer for 20-25 minutes until the lentils are tender.

4. Add salt and pepper to your liking.

Snack:

• Greek yogurt with honey and toasted hazelnuts.

Juice:

• Beetroot and carrot juice

DAY THREE

Breakfast: Berry Smoothie Bowl

• **INGREDIENTS**:

1 cup of assorted berries, including raspberries, blueberries, and strawberries

o One chilled banana

o 1/2 cup of spinach

o 1/2 cup of almond milk

o Granola, sliced banana, and chia seeds are the recommended toppings.

• *PREPARATION:*

1. In a blender, incorporate almond milk, thawed banana, spinach, and assorted berries.

2. Blend until the mixture is velvety and smooth.

3. Transfer the mixture to a vessel and garnish with granola, sliced bananas, and chia seeds.

Lunch: Stuffed bell peppers with quinoa

• **INGREDIENTS**:

2 bell peppers, seeded and divided

o One cup of prepared quinoa

o One can of black beans, strained and rinsed

o 1/2 cup of maize kernels

o 1/2 cup of salsa

O 1/2 teaspoon of cardamom

o Add salt and pepper to taste

- PREPARATION:

1. Turn the oven on to 375°F, or 190°C.

2. Combine cooked quinoa, black beans, maize, salsa, cumin, salt, and pepper in a basin.

3. Stuff the mixture into bell peppers that have been halved.

4. Place the stuffed peppers on a baking dish and bake for 25-30 minutes until they are tender.

- **INGREDIENTS**:

o Two chicken breasts

o Two tablespoons of olive oil

o One lemon, juiced and zested

o Two minced garlic cloves

o One teaspoon of dried oregano

o One teaspoon of dried thyme

o Add salt and pepper to taste

o. Chopped vegetables, including zucchini, bell peppers, and red onion

• *PREPARATION.*

1. Combine garlic, lemon zest, lemon juice, oregano, thyme, salt, and pepper in a basin. Whisk until well combined.

2. Marinate chicken breasts in the mixture for a minimum of 30 minutes.

3. Preheat the grill to medium-high fire.

4. Grill poultry for 6-8 minutes on each side until it is fully cooked.

5. Combine diced vegetables with olive oil, salt, and pepper.

6. Roast vegetables in the oven at 400°F (200°C) for 20-25 minutes until they are tender.

Snack:

• Cucumber slices with tzatziki dressing.

Juice:

• Ginger and orange juice

DAY FOUR:

Breakfast: Oatmeal with Almond Butter and Banana

• **INGREDIENTS**:

o 1/2 cup of dried oats

o One cup of almond milk

o One tablespoon of almond butter

o One split mature banana

o One tablespoon of honey

• PREPARATION:

1. Bring almond milk to a simmer in a saucepan.

2. Add the rolled oats and continue cooking for 5-7 minutes until the mixture thickens.

3. Transfer the oatmeal to a basin and garnish with almond butter, sliced bananas, and honey.

Lunch: Grilled Shrimp with Greek Salad

• INGREDIENTS:

o One cup of assorted greens

o 1/2 cucumber, cut

o. Half a cup of cherry tomatoes

o One-quarter cup of Kalamata olives

o 1/4 cup of shredded feta cheese

o Six prawns that have been broiled

o Two tablespoons of olive oil

o One teaspoonful of red wine vinegar

o One teaspoon of dried oregano

• *PREPARATION*:

1. Combine feta cheese, cherry tomatoes, cucumber, Kalamata olives, and assorted greens in a basin.

2. Add seared prawns to the top.

3. Sprinkle dried oregano and drizzle with red wine vinegar and olive oil.

Dinner: Vegetable Stir-Fry with Tofu

• **INGREDIENTS**:

o One cubed block of tofu

o Two teaspoons of soy sauce

o One tablespoon of sesame oil

o Two minced garlic cloves

o One teaspoon of minced ginger

o. Sliced vegetables, including broccoli, carrots, snap peas, and bell peppers

- Brown rice that has been cooked and is ready to serve

• *PREPARATION:*

1. Marinate tofu cubes in sesame oil and soy sauce in a basin.

2. Heat a large skillet or wok over medium-high heat.

3. Stir-fry for one minute with grated ginger and minced garlic.

4. Stir-fry the tofu until it turns golden brown.

5. Stir-fry a variety of vegetables until they are tender-crisp.

6. Serve with brown rice that has been prepared.

DAY FIVE:

INGREDIENTS

o One-quarter cup of chia seeds

o One cup of almond milk

• One tablespoon of maple syrup

o 1/2 teaspoon of vanilla extract

• *PREPARATION:*

1. Whisk almond milk, maple syrup, vanilla extract, and chia seeds in a basin.

2. Cover the container and place it in the refrigerator for the night.

3. Garnish with diced banana or fresh cherries.

Lunch: Turkey and Avocado Wrap

• **INGREDIENTS**:

o One whole-grain tortilla

o Three slices of turkey breast

o One-quarter avocado, diced

o A handful of spinach fronds

o One teaspoonful of hummus

• PREPARATION:

1. Spread hummus over the tortilla and place it flat.

2. Arrange spinach leaves, avocado, and turkey slices in a layer.

3. Twist the roll securely and then cut it in half.

Dinner: Baked Cod with Roasted Potatoes and Green Beans

• INGREDIENTS:

o Two cod fillets

o Two tablespoons of olive oil

o One lemon, freshly squeezed

o Two minced garlic cloves

o One teaspoon of preserved chives

o Add salt and pepper to taste

o Four medium-sized potatoes, divided

o One cup of green legumes

• **PREPARATION:**

1. Set oven temperature to 400°F, or 200°C.

2. Place cod fillets on a roasting tray.

3. Whisk together olive oil, lemon juice, minced garlic, dried dill, salt, and pepper in a small basin.

4. Distribute the mixture over the cod fillets.

5. Arrange green carrots and diced potatoes around the cod.

6. Bake for 20-25 minutes until the salmon is fully cooked and the potatoes are tender.

Snack:

• Rice pastries topped with banana slices and almond butter.

Juice:

• Mint and Watermelon Juice

DAY SIX:

Breakfast: Omelet with Feta and Spinach

• **INGREDIENTS**:

o Two eggs

o 1/4 cup of finely sliced spinach

o Two teaspoons of shredded feta cheese

o Add salt and pepper to taste

• PREPARATION:

1. Whisk together eggs, minced spinach, salt, and pepper in a basin.

2. Pour the egg mixture into a non-stick skillet that has been heated over medium heat.

3. Sprinkle feta cheese over one-half of the omelet after cooking until the margins are set.

4. Fold the remaining half over the cheese and continue cooking for an additional minute until the cheese has melted.

Lunch: Lentil and Vegetable Soup

• **INGREDIENTS**:

o One cup of drained dried legumes

o One diced onion

o Two carrots, cut

o Two minced celery stalks

o Four pints of vegetable broth

o One can of diced tomatoes

o One teaspoon of dried thyme

o Add salt and pepper to taste

• *PREPARATION:*

1. Sauté celery, carrots, and onion in a substantial saucepan until they are tender.

2. Add minced tomatoes, vegetable broth, lentils, and dried thyme.

3. Bring the mixture to a boil, then reduce the heat and allow it to simmer for 20-25 minutes until the lentils are tender.

4. Adjust the salt and pepper to taste.

- **INGREDIENTS**:

o One cup of prepared quinoa

o. Chopped barbecued vegetables, including zucchini, eggplant, bell peppers, and mushrooms

o 1/4 cup of shredded feta cheese

o Two tablespoons of balsamic vinaigrette

o Garnish with fresh basil fronds

- *PREPARATION:*

1. Add cooked quinoa, grilled vegetables, and crumbled feta cheese to a large bowl.

2. Drizzle the balsamic vinaigrette over the salad and toss to incorporate.

3. As a garnish, add some fresh basil leaves.

Snack:

• Peanut butter-covered celery stalks.

Juice:

• Turmeric, ginger, and carrot juice

DAY SEVEN:

Breakfast: Greek Yogurt Parfait

• **INGREDIENTS**:

o One cup of Greek yogurt

1/4 cup of cereal

o 1/4 cup of assorted fruit

o One tablespoon of honey

• *PREPARATION:*

1. Layer Greek yogurt, granola, and assorted berries in a glass.

2. Use honey to drizzle.

Caprese Salad for Lunch

• **INGREDIENTS**:

o One large tomato, cut

o One divided block of fresh mozzarella cheese

o Basil leaves that are freshly harvested

o Two tablespoons of balsamic marinade

o Add salt and pepper to taste

• *PREPARATION:*

1. Arrange segments of mozzarella and tomato on a platter.

2. Insert fresh basil leaves between the segments.

3. Season with salt and pepper and drizzle with balsamic marinade.

• **INGREDIENTS**:

o Two minced chicken breasts

o Two cups of diced assorted vegetables, including broccoli, cauliflower, and carrots

o One tablespoon of olive oil

o One teaspoon of Italian seasoning

o Add salt and pepper to taste

1/4 cup of minced Parmesan cheese

• *PREPARATION:*

1. Preheat the oven to 375°F (190°C).

2. Toss diced chicken and assorted vegetables with olive oil, Italian seasoning, salt, and pepper in a baking dish.

3. Sprinkle grated Parmesan cheese over the dish.

4. Bake for 25-30 minutes until the chicken is fully cooked and the vegetables are tender.

Snack:

• Trail blend consisting of dehydrated fruit, nuts, and seeds.

Juice:

• Apple juice, kale, and cucumber

A diverse array of flavors and nutrients is provided daily to promote a healthy diet. This includes beverages and munchies for hydration and energy. I hope you enjoy your meals!

CHAPTER EIGHT

Seven Desserts Procedural Recipes For Chronic Lymphocytic Leukemia

Chronic lymphocytic leukemia (CLL) is a form of malignancy that impacts the bone marrow and blood. During treatment, the management of diet can be essential for the promotion of overall health and well-being. Although the consumption of sugary, high-fat delicacies may be prohibited, there are still numerous nutritious and delectable alternatives to satiate one's sweet tooth.

Seven dessert recipes that are compatible with a CLL-friendly diet are presented below, with an emphasis on ingredients that enhance immunity, supply antioxidants, and sustain energy levels.

1. CHIA PUDDING WITH BERRIES

COMPONENTS:

• Two cups of almond milk

• 1/2 cup of chia seeds

• One cup of a combination of berries, including blueberries, raspberries, and strawberries

• 1 teaspoon of vanilla extract

• 1-2 tablespoons of maple syrup or honey (optional)

STEPS:

1. Combine almond milk, chia seeds, and vanilla extract in a basin.

2. Stir the mixture thoroughly to ensure that the chia seeds are evenly distributed.

3. After allowing it to settle for approximately five minutes, agitate it once more to prevent clumping.

4. Cover the basin and place it in the refrigerator for a minimum of four hours or overnight.

5. Blend half of the berries and incorporate them into the pudding before serving.

6. If desirable, garnish with the remaining fruit and a drizzle of honey or maple syrup.

2. Chocolate Avocado Mousse

COMPONENTS:

• Two mature avocados

• 1/4 cup of cocoa powder

• 1/4 cup of almond milk

• 1/4 cup of maple syrup or honey

• 1 teaspoon of vanilla extract

STEPS:

1. Place the avocado flesh in a blender.

2. Add almond milk, vanilla extract, honey or maple syrup, and cocoa powder.

3. Blend until the mixture is velvety and smooth.

4. Spoon the mixture into serving dishes and refrigerate for a minimum of 30 minutes before serving.

3. Quinoa with Apple Cinnamon

COMPONENTS:

• One cup of quinoa

• Two pints of water

• Two pears, cut

• One teaspoon of cinnamon

• 1/4 cup of raisins

• One tablespoon of maple syrup or honey

STEPS:

1. Rinse the quinoa with cool water.

2. Combine water and quinoa in a saucepan. Bring the mixture to a boil, then reduce the heat to a simmer and continue cooking for approximately 15 minutes, or until the water has been absorbed.

3. Incorporate diced apples, cinnamon, raisins, and honey or maple syrup into the prepared quinoa.

4. Stir the mixture thoroughly and allow it to settle for a few minutes to allow the flavors to meld.

5. Serve either at room temperature or refrigerated.

COMPONENTS:

• Four mature pears

• 1/4 cup of chopped walnuts

• Two tablespoons of honey

• One teaspoon of minced cinnamon

STEPS:

1. Set the oven's temperature to 175°C/350°F.

2. Divide the pears in half and remove the interior.

3. Arrange the pear halves on a baking tray.

4. Add sliced walnuts, moisten with honey, and sprinkle with cinnamon.

5. Bake for 20-25 minutes, or until the pears are soft.

6. Arrange for a heated serving.

5. Almonds and Pomegranate in Greek Yogurt

COMPONENTS:

• Two cups of Greek yogurt

• 1/2 cup of pomegranate seeds

• 1/4 cup of sliced almonds

• One tablespoon of maple syrup or honey

STEPS:

1. Distribute Greek yogurt among serving dishes.

2. Sprinkle sliver almonds and pomegranate seeds on top.

3. Drizzle with maple syrup or honey.

4. Serve immediately.

COMPONENTS:

• Three mature mangoes

• One cup of coconut milk

• One tablespoon of citrus juice

• 2 tablespoons of maple syrup or honey (optional)

STEPS:

1. Mangoes should be peeled and diced.

2. Mangoes, coconut milk, lime juice, and honey or maple syrup should be combined in a blender.

3. Blend until the mixture is uniform.

4. Transfer the mixture to a freezer-safe container and freeze for a minimum of four hours.

5. Scoop and serve.

COMPONENTS:

• Two mature avocados

• 1 cup rolled oats

• 1/4 cup dark chocolate morsels (optional)

• 1 teaspoon of vanilla extract

STEPS:

1. Preheat the oven to 350°F (175°C).

2. In a basin, puree the bananas until smooth.

3. Add rolled cereals, chocolate morsels (if using), and vanilla extract. Mix well.

4. Spoonfuls of the mixture should be dropped onto a parchment paper-lined baking sheet.

5. Bake for 15-20 minutes, or until cookies are golden brown.

6. Let chill on a wire rack before serving.

Dietary Guidelines For CLL

1. Focus on Whole Foods: Emphasize fruits, vegetables, whole cereals, lean proteins, and healthy fats.

2. Limit Sugar and Processed Foods: These can impair the immune system and contribute to unwanted weight gain.

3. Stay Hydrated: Drink plenty of water and avoid sugary beverages.

4. Balance Protein and Carbs: Ensure a healthy balance to maintain energy levels without blood sugar surges.

5. Antioxidant-Rich Foods: Include berries, verdant greens, almonds, and seeds to combat oxidative stress.

6. Healthy Fats: Incorporate sources like avocados, olive oil, and almonds for anti-inflammatory benefits.

7. Moderate Portions: Keep portion sizes reasonable to maintain a healthy weight.

By integrating these dessert recipes into your diet, you can enjoy delectable delights that align with the nutritional requirements of someone managing CLL.

CHAPTER NINE

Seven Smoothies For Chronic Lymphocytic Leukemia: Recipes And Guidelines

Chronic lymphocytic leukemia (CLL) is a form of malignancy that impacts the bone marrow and blood. A well-balanced diet can play a supportive role in managing CLL, and smoothies are an excellent way to incorporate nutrient-dense foods into your diet.

Here are seven smoothie recipes tailored to support CLL patients, followed by dietary guidelines to optimize their benefits.

1. GREEN POWER SMOOTHIE

COMPONENTS:

• 1 cup spinach

• 1/2 cucumber

• 1 green apple

• 1/2 avocado

• 1 teaspoonful of chia seeds

• 1 cup unadulterated almond milk

• One tablespoon of honey (optional)

STEPS:

1. Wash all raw ingredients thoroughly.

2. Peel and slice the cucumber, apple, and avocado.

3. All ingredients should be combined in a blender.

4. Blend until the mixture is uniform.

5. Serve immediately.

COMPONENTS:

• 1 cup assorted berries (blueberries, strawberries, raspberries)

• 1/2 cup plain Greek yogurt

• 1 tablespoon flaxseeds

• 1 cup water or coconut water

• One tablespoon of honey (optional)

STEPS:

1. Rinse the cherries.

2. Combine all components in the blender.

3. Blend until the mixture is smooth and velvety.

4. Take pleasure in a calm state.

COMPONENTS:

• One cup of pineapple slices

• One-half of a mango

• One orange (segmented and skinned)

• One-half cup of carrot juice

• 1 tablespoon of minced ginger

• 1/2 cup of coconut water or water

STEPS:

1. Mango and pineapple should be peeled and chopped.

2. Combine all components in the blender.

3. Blend until the ingredients are thoroughly integrated.

4. Serve immediately.

COMPONENTS:

• One banana

• 1/2 cup of almond butter

• One tablespoon of flaxseeds

• One cup of strained almond milk

• One teaspoon of cinnamon

• One teaspoon of honey (optional)

STEPS:

1. Slice the banana after it has been peeled.

2. All ingredients should be combined in a blender.

3. Blend until the mixture is velvety and smooth.

4. Pour the beverage into a glass and savor it.

COMPONENTS:

• One grapefruit (segmented and trimmed)

• One orange (segmented and skinned)

• Juiced half of a lemon

• One tablespoon of chia seeds

• One cup of coconut water

• One tablespoon of honey (optional)

STEPS:

1. Peel and segment the grapefruit and orange.

2. Combine all components in the blender.

3. Blend until the mixture is uniform.

4. Serve immediately.

COMPONENTS:

• One small beet, skinned and sliced

• One cup of a combination of berries, including blueberries, strawberries, and raspberries

• One-half of a banana

• One tablespoon of chia seeds

• One cup of water or coconut water

STEPS:

1. Prepare the beet by peeling and chopping it.

2. Combine all components in the blender.

3. Blend until the mixture is uniform.

4. Take pleasure in a calm state.

COMPONENTS:

• One-half of an avocado

• One cup of kale

• One-half of a green apple

• One-half of a cucumber

• One tablespoon of flaxseeds

• One cup of strained almond milk

STEPS:

1. Thoroughly rinse all fresh ingredients.

2. Chop the cucumber, apple, and avocado.

3. Combine all components in the blender.

4. Blend until the mixture is velvety and smooth.

5. Serve immediately.

Dietary Recommendations For Chronic Lymphoma

1. Foods that are abundant in nutrients:

o Concentrate on fruits and vegetables, particularly those that are rich in antioxidants, such as cruciferous vegetables, verdant greens, and berries.

o Incorporate nutritious lipids from sources such as avocados, almonds, seeds, and olive oil.

2. Hydration:

o Ensure that you consume an adequate amount of fluids, to consume a minimum of eight glasses of water each day. Coconut water can serve as a nutritious and hydrating alternative.

3. Protein:

o Incorporate plant-based protein sources, such as tempeh and tofu, as well as lean proteins like chicken, fish, and legumes.

o Smoothies may be supplemented with Greek yogurt and nut butter to increase their protein content.

4. Fiber:

o To promote digestive health, incorporate foods that are high in fiber. Smoothies are an excellent method for incorporating fruits, vegetables, chia seeds, and flaxseeds into one's diet to increase fiber intake.

5. Refrain from consuming processed foods:

o Reduce consumption of unhealthy lipids, refined carbohydrates, and processed foods.

Emphasize the consumption of whole, unprocessed nutrients to promote overall health.

6. Immune Support:

o The immune system can be bolstered by foods that are high in selenium, zinc, and vitamins C and E. Leafy greens, almonds, seeds, and citrus fruits are all excellent options.

7. Consult with healthcare providers:

o Before making substantial dietary modifications, it is crucial to seek the advice of a healthcare provider or nutritionist, particularly if you are currently receiving treatment for CLL.

By integrating these guidelines and smoothie recipes into your daily regimen, you can promote your overall well-being and nutritional requirements while managing Chronic Lymphocytic Leukemia.

CHAPTER TEN

Grocery Shopping And Meal Planning

Formulating A Weekly Meal Plan

Begin by compiling a list of the meals you will consume on each day of the week, which should include breakfast, lunch, supper, and refreshments. Concentrate on a well-rounded diet that includes a diverse array of vegetables, lean proteins, whole cereals, and healthy lipids. For instance, oatmeal for breakfast, grilled chicken salad for lunch, and roasted salmon with quinoa for dinner could all be part of a Monday regimen.

Creating A Shopping List

List all necessary ingredients after your meal plan is completed. Arrange the inventory according to categories such as cereals, meat, dairy, and produce. For instance, if your strategy involves a chicken stir-fry, incorporate chicken, broccoli, bell peppers, soy sauce, and brown rice into your shopping list.

Strategies For Efficient Grocery Shopping

Begin by perusing the perimeter of the store, which is typically where fresh produce, dairy, and meat are situated. To mitigate impulse purchases, refrain from purchasing when you are famished. Utilize your grocery list to maintain focus and contemplate purchasing in-season produce for superior quality and pricing.

Freezing And Batch Cooking Meals

Commit a few hours each week to the preparation of significant quantities of meals. Divide them into individual servings and freeze them for convenient, nutritious meals throughout the week. For example, prepare a substantial quantity of chili, portion it into containers, and freeze them for effortless reheating.

Minimizing Food Waste

Plan dishes that incorporate comparable ingredients to prevent overconsumption. For instance, the following day, incorporate the remaining roasted vegetables into a broth or salad. To extend the shelf life of perishable items, it is important to store them properly. Additionally, to prevent food waste, it is important to be inventive with any remnants.

Conclusion

Although a Chronic Lymphocytic Leukemia (CLL) diet is not a panacea, it can significantly contribute to the overall health and well-being of individuals with CLL, potentially enhancing their outcomes. It is imperative to prioritize a diet that is abundant in fruits, vegetables, whole cereals, lean proteins, and healthy lipids. These foods are a source of essential vitamins, minerals, and antioxidants that can enhance the immune system and assist in the prevention of the negative consequences of cancer and its treatment.

Inflammation can be reduced and metabolic health can be improved by reducing the consumption of processed foods, carbohydrates, and red meats. This may alleviate certain symptoms and enhance quality of life. Additionally, maintaining a balanced intake of nutrients and remaining hydrated can assist in the management of fatigue and the maintenance of overall energy levels.

Personalized dietary recommendations that are customized to the unique requirements and treatment plans of the individual can be obtained by consulting with a dietitian who specializes in oncology nutrition. Although CLL cannot be treated through diet alone, it is a valuable element of a comprehensive disease management strategy.

In summary, individuals with CLL can improve their quality of life, support their treatment regimen, and enhance their health by implementing a nutritious and balanced diet. This integrative approach underscores the significance of nutrition as a supportive therapy in the comprehensive management of chronic lymphocytic leukemia.

THE END